HOW I LOST 36,000 POUNDS

This book represents the conclusions reached after eighteen years of experience as a practicing physician

Distributed by

JanAn Enterprises
P.O. Box 49005
Los Angeles, California, 90049

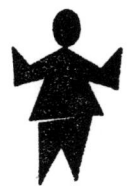

HOW I LOST 36,000 POUNDS

A PRACTICAL APPROACH TO WEIGHT REDUCTION

by Melvin Anchell, M.D.

1964

HARLO PRESS   DETROIT, MICH.

© MELVIN ANCHELL, M.D. 1964

All rights reserved, including the right to reproduce this book or any portions thereof in any form.

Library of Congress Catalog Card Number: 64-23142

PRINTED BY
HARLO PRESS

16854 Hamilton Avenue   Detroit, Michigan 48203

DEDICATED

TO

JOHN McGRAW, M.D.

CONTENTS...

	Introduction	9
1.	Meat for Life and Why	15
2.	The Meat Diet	21
3.	Dietary Amnesia	31
4.	Appetite Killers	35
5.	Two Kinds of Hunger	39
6.	Abnormal Hunger	43
7.	A Magic Way	47
8.	Overweight and Disease	51
9.	The Cholesterol Craze	57
10.	Your Best Friends Are Your Worst Enemies	63
11.	Eating for Beauty	67
12.	Weight Charts	71
13.	Obesity in Children	73
14.	What about Milk?	79
15.	The Hungry Anonymous	85
16.	Life without Food	87
17.	Modification of the Meat Diet	89
18.	Dear Doctor	91
19.	Some Must Remain Fat	95
	Cases	105

INTRODUCTION . . .

SIX SHOATS AND A 68-YEAR-OLD MAN TAUGHT ME that I was overweight. My neighbor, who was not only elderly, but an alcoholic, was still chipper after helping me round up six run-a-way young pigs while I had to take to my bed to recuperate. At first I thought malaria contracted in World War II was responsible for my shortness of breath and my heart flutterings. I envisioned having to give up the little farm with which I was experimenting as a recreational side-line to my practice of general medical practitioner. But in diagnosing myself,

How I Lost 36,000 Pounds

I realized that I must blame life-long eating habits which inevitably led to obesity.

Members of my family were ice-cream eaters. No day was complete without its visit to the confectionary and a side trip on the way home to pick up something special from the bake shop. The Greek proprietors of the confectionary were almost like members of the family; we visited them so often. They were masters at concocting sundaes, luscious with fudge sauce, and finally retired, I am convinced, with a fine nest egg saved from our purchases alone.

When one of the children of the family was unhappy, my grandmother's invariable remedy was homemade chocolate cake. Since her death such cake can be found only in Heaven. My solicitous mother stuffed us regularly with other goodies to the point that my sister, a handsome girl, constantly fought unsuccessfully to keep her weight down. Food was one of the big pleasures of our lives. No morphine addict liked his narcotic better than we liked our chocolate cake. Now I was paying the penalty.

I was determined to get rid of that fat, and I set about it the best way I knew. My training and experience

Introduction

included dealing with patients whose health demanded that they reduce.

Some of them had heart conditions, some were diabetic, others had hypertension, but most just wanted to look better. For each I had prescribed low calorie diets, the standard practice of the times. Now I had to prescribe for myself and to take my own medicine—unappetizing, starvation meals.

I had learned that some patients, even with life itself at stake, would not remain on the diets I prescribed. I came to learn the hard way that no tranquilizer equals the soothing effect of a big piece of chocolate cake. But I put myself on a low calorie diet, and in three weeks I had lost about ten pounds; in six weeks I had gained it back with four additional pounds. It was impossible to stay on such a diet and to do the work of a busy, general practitioner on call twenty-four hours a day.

Such experiences are common to most people troubled with the slightest tendency toward obesity. Probably the first fat merchant who appealed for advice was told to copy his poorer neighbor and eat that neighbor's restricted diet. This was the first starvation (low calorie) diet. And probably the fat merchant, like most of his descendants, found the advice impossible to take. Of the many patients for whom I have prescribed low calorie diets, not one was able to make a permanent adjustment to such a diet, an adjustment that would make the weight loss permanent.

In short, one can't lose weight by starving without losing life itself by dying of malnutrition. Yet a dieter who stops dieting inevitably gains back the weight he lost, usually with a few pounds extra. To tell a man to starve himself indefinitely is like telling an alcoholic to take one drink and to leave the bottle on the table. It can't be done.

As for myself, after three months of the most intense effort, accompanied by nagging hunger most of the time, I was ready to give up and just be fat; when in through the mail came one of my scientific journals reporting new findings in the field of nutrition.

This book represents the application of new findings in medicine, first to my own body and second, for the past ten years, to the bodies of innumerable patients who have successfully solved their obesity problems by means of the methods outlined in the following pages. I learned the hard way and passed on to my patients what I have learned.

Introduction

I HAD LEARNED THAT:

You can't lose weight permanently by starving.

If you lose weight temporarily by starving, you'll gain it back, often with added pounds.

Starvation is malnutrition.

A low calorie diet is starvation.

MEAT FOR LIFE AND WHY

CHAPTER ONE

THE PHYSIOLOGY DEPARTMENT OF A LARGE MEDICAL school in the United States in the early 1950's published the results of intensive studies of the action and effects of a meat (protein and fat) diet on the body. Their findings were revolutionary. They discovered that a man could eat as much meat as he wanted, and that within a comparatively short period his body would find its natural and most healthful weight.

Clinical experience with thousands of patients since this time reveals that this fact cannot be disputed. Regardless of the condition or age of the patient, regardless of whether he is thin or obese, or whether he is sick or healthy, meat is the food he will improve on.

Meat is made up of protein and fat. From these two substances the body makes the building blocks and creates the energy it needs. The body is like a wonderful chemical laboratory which converts these substances even into sugar if the body needs it.

Fat is the major fuel for the body. As soon as this substance reaches the body cells, it is immediately and completely utilized and oxidized by these cells. The fat is converted into sugar: part of it is used, and the excess is converted in the liver into glycogen, where it is stored until the body needs it. When the body needs quick fuel, it is called forth from the liver; the glycogen is converted into a simpler sugar and utilized for energy.

When carbohydrates (sugars) are taken into the body, this normal body process is disrupted. The body may utilize some of this sugar as energy. The rest of it, however, or the fat which would have been used as fuel, is converted into excess body fat.

Protein is almost entirely absorbed by the body but never is deposited as excess fat. And oddly enough, when

Meat for Life and Why

fats are eaten, abnormal body fat is burned up faster by the action of the proteins and fat. A man can eat as much meat as he likes without getting fat. Furthermore, he will never get too thin on such a diet. A meat diet establishes an ideal chemical balance and weight in the body.

Prehistoric men were hunters and meat eaters. They did not suffer away their lives with diabetes, high blood pressure, gall bladder disease, and other debilitating conditions. They lived vigorously and actively; they had to be extremely strong to survive and to ward off the diseases associated with contaminated food and water, with injuries, and with other infections such as tuberculosis. There were no wonder drugs or operating rooms with surgeons available.

As ages passed, and man began to learn how to control his environment, he also learned to keep his food supply in his backyard by growing it from the ground rather than by hunting for it. His food-growing was invaluable to him in attaining civilization. The only trouble was that his digestive system did not keep pace with his cultural achievements. Man's organs remained appropriate for the intake of meat. The eating of grain and other products grown from the soil satisfied his taste buds but confused his body's chemical laboratory. The body did not know how to utilize these other foods (grains, vegetables, fruits, sugars, and other carbohydrates).

The body utilizes these new foods to its capacity but is unable completely to digest and to burn up these materials to the end products. More of these foods, consequently, must be eaten to supply the energy that an equivalent amount of meat would provide. Most foods that are grown form large amounts of residue whereas meat is almost completely digested when it goes through the digestive system.

Meat is utilized in the body to provide the building material for new tissue such as muscle, for blood, for bone, for heart, etc. These structures are built of protein and fat, and they derive their energy from sugar. The meat not used for building material is converted by the body into sugar for energy. If too much meat is eaten by an individual, his body takes what it needs for building and energy purposes and then completely breaks down what is left over into end products which are readily excreted from the kidneys, lungs, sweat glands, and intestines. The body knows its own needs and when given the proper food (meat) will maintain itself in a perfect state of equilibrium, neither too fat nor too thin.

Meat for Life and Why

If, on the other hand, grown foods such as grains, etc., are eaten, some digestion does occur, but large residues of this type of food remain undigested. What is absorbed into the blood stream is only partially metabolized. The body cannot build itself from such foods, for they are primarily carbohydrates which cannot be converted into proteins, the body building blocks. Carbohydrates are broken down into simple and complex sugars and, as such, supply energy, but if too much carbohydrate is eaten, the only thing that the body can do with it is to store it as fat, excess fat, unneeded fat, the kind of fat that is a slow cancer.

When man first stopped hunting for his food, he learned to herd and to tend his game in order to have food close by, allowing him the convenience and safety of living in larger groups and villages. Eventually, he not only herded the animals he used for food, but he began to emulate their eating habits. He found he liked the taste of food from the soil as well as from the hoof, and as civilization progressed he surpassed his teachers, the herbivorous animals, and used a multitude of foods which he grew. The only thing wrong was that he did not have the stomach of a cow and could not properly digest or assimilate the cow's food.

Furthermore, as man learned to enjoy eating for its own sake, he not only ate to keep alive, but established this function of the body as a pastime, a pleasure, a social grace, and a status symbol. Food became associated with man's social, even with his spiritual activities.

But eating is the only vital bodily function in which man participates beyond his needs. For example, we need to breathe to keep alive, but we never gulp down excessive quantities of air. We let the body set the pace. We could do the same with food.

Following is the meat diet. It must be remembered concerning this diet that it must be followed implicitly. A crumb of any food not listed on the diet, even a sugar-coated medicinal tablet, will act as a catalyst to convert the whole of the food taken into fat, much as a thimbleful of tetraethyl lead converts the burning qualities of a gallon of regular gasoline. A crumb of stuffing, the breading on cutlets, Worcestershire Sauce or ketchup, meat tenderizer, literally a crumb of floured gravy, will make the diet a fattening instead of a thinning one.

THE MEAT DIET

CHAPTER TWO

BREAKFAST, LUNCH AND DINNER ARE OF THE SAME TYPE. You eat three big meals a day and lose seven pounds or more of excess weight a month.

FIRST COURSE OF EACH MEAL: One-half pound or more of fresh meat with the fat. This part of the diet is unlimited. You may eat as much as you wish. Most of the meat you buy is not fat enough; extra fat is advisable. Good meats are roast beef, steak, roast lamb, lamb chops, stew, fresh pork and pork chops. Hamburger is acceptable if ground just before it is cooked.

How I Lost 36,000 Pounds

Season the meat with black pepper before it is cooked or use paprika, celery seed, lemon, chopped parsley or celery tops.

Do not use foods containing salt, such as soup, bacon, smoked ham, canned fish, frankfurters, bologna, canned or spiced meat, or salted butter.

SECOND COURSE OF EACH MEAL: This part of the diet is limited. At each meal you have a choice of an ordinary portion of any one of the following:

- White Potatoes
- Sweet Potatoes
- Half Grapefruit
- Bunch of Grapes
- Slice of Melon
- Banana or Pear
- Raspberries or Blueberries

At the end of each meal have a cup of black coffee or clear tea without sugar. Do not use saccharine. Your only other beverage is half a lemon in a glass of water. Weight must be regulated completely to normal before other foods can be added or you will quickly regain the weight you have lost.

NOTE PARTICULARLY that this diet contains no bread, flour, sugar, or alcohol.

The Meat Diet

Those dieters wishing to lose with extra rapidity may eliminate salt for a few weeks from this diet since salt tends to hold water in the body. The eating of additional fat will also contribute to a quicker weight loss. It should be remembered, however, that water is not fat, and is never fattening; it never contributes to the deposit of excess fatty tissues. Water may be drunk at will. The diet will be more palatable, of course, if salt is added.

Alcohol, as such, cannot be converted into fat, nor into work energy. It does, however, contribute body heat which in turn leaves fat deposits unused which otherwise might be destroyed to create needed energy. Dieters who feel they must drink are advised to drink in limited amounts sugar-free alcoholic drinks, using gin, whiskey, or vodka with carbonated or plain water, rather than wines, beer, egg-nog, or cocktails made with any sugar substance such as ginger ale.

After three weeks of any change in food habits, a person may feel painfully deprived and, like a starving prisoner of war, may dream of forbidden foods. A chocolate ice-cream soda or a piece of apple pie may prove irresistible. If the new eating habits can be sustained in spite of a temporary lapse, they will become fairly firmly established, and the person can go on for months in spite of a tendency toward occasional indiscretions which can be more and more easily resisted. The longer the new eating habits are sustained, the more palatable and satisfying the meat meals will become.

When the body has attained its individual norm, not its chart weight but its own proper weight, weight loss ceases, and then this diet can be modified by the addition of certain foods to be found in the modification chart. The modified diet is a maintenance diet and will not cause weight loss.

QUESTIONS

1. What happens if I substitute other foods of approximately the same chemical content as the diet foods listed?

    ANSWER: You won't lose that week, and all your deprivation will be for nothing. This is a diet in which no substitutes should be made.

2. What about vitamins? Won't I need Vitamin C?

    ANSWER: Meat is a complete food; lions and tigers do not run to the grocery store for their Vitamin C. Anyway, Vitamin C is contained in grapefruit, pears, and berries, all foods on the diet.

The Meat Diet

3. Isn't this diet very expensive? Meat costs a lot.

   ANSWER: If you cut out the pies, cakes, breads, and soft drinks, you'll save enough to pay the butcher's bill. Besides meat is cheaper than the doctor or the undertaker.

4. What can I drink?

   ANSWER: Water is the only beverage natural to and beneficial to man after he is six months old.

5. Why can't I have saccharine?

   ANSWER: Because the quicker you lose your taste for sugar, the easier this diet will be for you. Remember, this is not merely a diet, it is a change of eating habits which will be beneficial to you your whole life long.

6. I have never been a meat eater, and I could not bear to eat meat for breakfast. What shall I do?

   ANSWER: After your ideal weight has been reached, you will have no problem, for the modified maintenance diet allows other foods. In the meantime, eat a portion of the fruit allowed on your diet and omit the meat for breakfast.

7. You say that I can have pork. Why can't I have ham or bacon or sausage?

    ANSWER: Ham and bacon are usually sugar cured and sausage contains sugar. Avoid them for this reason. Also avoid mashed potatoes that have been mixed with milk, and gravy that has been thickened with flour. Only natural gravy is acceptable.

8. If I lose weight, won't my skin sag?

    ANSWER: With the meat diet the body will, on the contrary, get firmer and the muscle tone will improve. The skin will develop resilience and elasticity and will fit snugly over the underlying structure.

9. Why don't you advocate exercise?

    ANSWER: A man must walk 35 miles to lose one pound. Besides, exercise increases the appetite. It does improve muscle-tone and will do no harm if you will stay on your diet.

10. Why can't I substitute cottage cheese for meat, or strawberries for blueberries, or beans for potatoes?

    ANSWER: The answer is simple. Because it won't work. If you must, try it and see.

The Meat Diet

11. You say that I cannot eat too much meat and fat. Can I eat too little?

    ANSWER: No; but the more fat you eat, the faster you will lose weight.

12. I have stayed on the diet completely for one week, yet I have not lost weight. What is the matter?

    ANSWER: If you have not eaten one crumb of any other substance except what was listed on the diet, check the labels for dextrose, or glucose, or sugar. Did you take a pill that contained sugar? Did you chew gum? Any of these things will affect your weight loss. If you did not do any one of these, check your scales; you'll find you have lost weight.

    Remember, the pleasure of eating a piece of pie lasts only a few seconds, but will spoil your record of weight loss for a week.

13. I can't drink coffee without sugar. What shall I do?

    ANSWER: After nine or ten days of coffee without sugar you will not like coffee *with* sugar.

14. I tried that and now I don't like coffee. What shall I do?

ANSWER: Drink tea or water. But remember, three cups of coffee will kill your appetite for food, temporarily at least.

15. Can I lose weight too fast?

ANSWER: This diet is a slow weight losing diet because it involves a change in eating habits, but it will never make you feel weak, as will a starvation diet.

16. Why can't I have a hamburger?

ANSWER: Stores and restaurants frequently add cereal and flavoring to the hamburger.

17. You say that excess body fat is parasitic and of no value. Isn't this fat an insulator?

ANSWER: Most fat people have poor heat regulating mechanisms, shivering in the winter and sweating in the summer.

18. Why are dogs used in studying the effects of medicine on the stomach?

ANSWER: Dogs are carniverous and the action and function of their stomachs closely resembles that of the human being.

The Meat Diet

19. If eating is such an integral part of man's adjustment to civilized living, what can be used to take the place of food?

    ANSWER: Until man learns better control of his anxieties and tensions, food will continue to be used by some for its tranquilizing properties. In some cases devotion to a hobby, participation in community projects, or other activities, whereby tense energy can be used, help. Even the use of prescribed tranquilizers is less injurious than overeating by indulging in fattening types of food. The meat diet does not add weight even though excessive quantities of it are eaten.

20. I am obese and have high blood pressure, but I cannot give up the food I love. What can I do?

    ANSWER: If life without the pleasure of the old foodstuffs is unbearable, and you can't control yourself long enough to adjust to new eating habits, then the best thing to do is eat and be happy. Longevity without happiness is not too great a reward under these circumstances.

21. How many patients on the meat diet have you closely followed?

    ANSWER: Over 2,000.

DIETARY

AMNESIA

CHAPTER THREE

"Don't tell me I've been eating anything! I haven't been eating anything and look at me!"

Mrs. X entered the consulting room, an accusing finger shaking almost under my nose. For a two-year period, like an alcoholic, Mrs. X had been on and off of a diet to lose weight. Her husband, she said, ate anything and everything while she maintained a restricted diet of her own devising and on it had gained back all the weight she had lost six months before.

Arguments are useless in such situations. To tell the patient she cannot gain weight from breathing air does no good. Even that rare thyroid condition which obese individuals always claim cannot cause obesity unless the person's intake of food is greater than can be used.

Mrs. X was convinced that her food intake was truly a starvation diet, and she went into detail concerning her daily menus, meals so impossibly meager that I wondered she had survived at all. Such statements by overweight patients are routine. Eating is such a firmly fixed habit, especially in the obese, that it is almost unconsciously done. As Mrs. X waddled through the door to the scales, an incoming patient proved to me that this was indeed the case with Mrs. X.

"Look at that!" said the new patient with a sniff of disapproval in her direction. "Isn't that terrible? And that woman comes in the drug store twice a day to eat the richest sundaes I can make." The incoming patient was the counter girl in the drug store down the street.

No wonder the scales revealed that Mrs. X had indeed gained back all the pounds she had lost when she was under my care six months before.

In the mind of Mrs. X these forays to the drugstore were as natural as drinking a glass of water and were quickly forgotten. I call this dietary amnesia. The

Dietary Amnesia

patient truly does not remember the food she consumes. Often her husband comes with her and affirms that she ate "no breakfast but a cup of coffee." He does not realize that fifteen minutes after his departure she begins a series of invasions of the icebox, justified because she "ate no breakfast."

At formal meals the dieter is aware that she is eating and rigidly controls herself both because she wishes to cooperate and because others are present and aware of the amount of food eaten. Between meals it is a different matter. Almost unconsciously, the dieter begins to nibble. First she drinks a glass of orange juice, remembering that she ate no breakfast. Then she has a piece of bread with butter and jelly. It is dry without a glass of milk. At ten she is still hungry, tired from carrying around her excess weight, and she eats a piece of pie left from dinner the night before and drinks another glass of milk. She justifies this because the amount of food adds up in her mind to one light meal.

Just as a baby needs to suck, Mrs. X and others like her truly need to put food into their mouths. It is hopeless and cruel to try to eradicate this habit. It cannot be done. For many such people, food supplies life's main pleasure or gratifies profound psychological needs.

For such individuals all diets that restrict food intake fail. But even these individuals can maintain normal and appropriate weight by a return to the food truly natural to man.

Mrs. X was reassured and encouraged to resume the eating habits which would bring weight loss and at the same time would allow her to gratify her real craving for quantities of food.

Eating or placing something in their mouths is such an integral part of the being of some individuals that the intake of food becomes a reflex. Such people cannot recall how many times they have eaten any more than a person can remember how many times he blinked his eyes.

Dietary amnesia is augmented by the sense of guilt an overweight person feels when he eats anything. Then he eats again to ease his increased tension.

Everybody thinks that the reason for his particular obesity is a metabolic deficiency, or an inherited defect, both of which are extremely rare, and neither of which would cause obesity without overeating. Others declare that they gain weight if they look at or smell food.

APPETITE KILLERS

CHAPTER FOUR

A 38-YEAR-OLD, 186-POUND NEIGHBOR, MRS. Y, CORNERED me in my office one day with the plea that she wanted to lose weight. Mrs. V, she said, who with her husband ran the neighborhood grocery store, was taking some kind of pills that helped her to lose weight. She wanted pills like that.

This is an old story. Everybody wants to get thin the easy way. The trouble is, pills will not make a person get thin. The usual prescription, probably one of the amphetamines, will help to cut the appetite for only about two weeks. After that, amphetamines supply energy but do not reduce the appetite. Furthermore, they can be dangerous.

At Mrs. Y's insistence I prescribed an amphetamine and wrote a prescription for a two-weeks' supply, hoping I could help her develop proper eating habits in that time. After that two weeks, I never saw Mrs. Y again professionally until she reappeared in my office nine months later. During this interval I had moved to a nearby city and set up practice there.

Mrs. Y was in a nervous twitch. When she came into the consultation room, her eyes were abnormally wide, and she could hardly sit still. The scales revealed that she had not lost a pound although she had lost about seven during the two weeks that I had seen her. She had not maintained the eating habits I had prescribed but had instead returned to her former foods, depending upon the pills to help her reduce their quantity. Her neighborhood druggist had obligingly refilled the prescription not realizing that he was contributing to what could be a real addiction; for addiction can develop as the result of these crutches.

Mrs. Y, however, a highly moral woman, when I warned her of the possibility of addiction, declared she

Appetite Killers

would never take another pill and resolved that she would battle her appetite in a more sensible way.

Amphetamines (Benzedrine and Dexedrine) are the most widely used drugs for weight loss. They may decrease the appetite for approximately fourteen days. After this period, the appetite-decreasing effect is lost, and the patient may continue to rely on these medicines because they make him feel more energetic and stimulated. These properties of the drug may lead to addiction, but I find that no additional weight loss will accrue.

It is my observation that patients lose weight for two weeks with any prescription, even with a sugar tablet, because during this length of time their determination is high to follow instructions and to reduce their weight. After two weeks their previous habits and their need for food as a solace for stress overcomes their determination.

Thyroid preparations should be used only by persons who have a deficiency of thyroid activity and should never be used as a diet-reducing aid. Patients taking thyroid often feel they have the magic ingredient that will make them thin. They then become careless about their eating with a resulting gain of weight.

Diuretics, another drug type often requested by misguided patients, reduces the quantity of water in the system and thereby achieves what might be called a false weight loss. The fatty tissues are in no sense reduced, and the patient in fact soon remedies his waterless condition by drinking more liquids. If he does not, his health may be damaged.

Exercise, too, is no weight remedy. A 250-pound man would have to climb twenty flights of stairs to rid himself of the effects of eating one slice of bread. A person can lose one pound of fat by walking thirty-five miles, providing he eats nothing on the way.

Cigarettes? Smoking to stop eating? All I can say is that I have never written a prescription for cigarettes.

Coffee is an ever available appetite killer. One cup of black coffee will not blot out the vision of a piece of apple pie; two cups of coffee will begin to do it, and three cups will satisfy sufficiently so that the keen desire for food is eliminated. The coffee must be taken black, and if the habit of drinking it black is cultivated for two weeks, cream and sugar with the coffee will not even be desired. The worse the coffee tastes, the better an appetite killer it will be. Tea and de-caffeinated coffee serve the purpose almost as well.

TWO
KINDS
OF HUNGER

CHAPTER FIVE

A LUMBERJACK GETS UP A BIT LATE ONE MORNING AND, after gulping a cup of coffee, rushes off to work without breakfast. He forgets his lunch pail. Since his work is far from home, he cannot come home for lunch, and by the time of his return in late afternoon he is ravenously hungry. Men doing work of this kind are probably the largest calorie users. Fortunately his wife, noticing that he went without his lunch, has prepared a big, three-pound steak and a baked potato for him. When he finishes eating this meal, he is satisfied.

How I Lost 36,000 Pounds

A housewife gets up in the morning to the usual stir of getting a husband off to work and children off to school. When the house is quiet, she begins her work, proud of the fact that at breakfast she has maintained the diet she began two days before.

At ten o'clock she discovers that the milkman has left the wrong kind of cottage cheese, and she is irritated. She gets just a little tense. At eleven o'clock her next-door neighbor calls to say that her dog has knocked over the neighbor's garbage can again. Our housewife feels both guilty and irritated. But she broils herself a hamburger patty for lunch and eats some grapes, feeling pleased that she is still on her diet and has eaten only a few more grapes than she was supposed to. At two-fifteen the children come home from school. They are quarreling. Johnny tells his mother that another little boy has torn his shirt. She feels she cannot stand all this confusion, and she gets a little more tense. But she drinks a cup of coffee and eats nothing.

At five, her husband comes home. He has had a hard day; his boss has given him an impossible job to do. He criticizes his wife because the children are noisy. He tells her she is a poor housekeeper. She becomes more tense but goes about getting dinner. She has prepared

Two Kinds of Hunger

steak and baked potatoes. She eats heavily but is not satisfied. Her hunger is not for calories but for tension relief.

Before she began her diet she was not conscious of tension. She ate to counteract her feelings of disturbance. When the wrong milk delivery was made, she would have another piece of toast with jelly and a cup of coffee with sugar and cream. When her neighbor complained, she would eat a few cookies from the cookie-jar. When her children quarreled, she would soothe herself with one of the peanut butter sandwiches she made for their after-school snack. When her husband complained, she would make each of them a cocktail and cheer herself still further with a rich dessert. The immediate pleasure from a few bites of sugar-rich food acted as a distraction from her troubles.

The pleasure of eating and the relief of tension revolve about food for many people. A removal of customary food intake leaves tension unrelieved, resulting in the greater expenditure of energy which in turn produces a feeling of weakness.

There are two types of hunger: first, the hunger for energy-producing calories, and secondly, the hunger for tension-relieving and pleasure-producing calories.

How I Lost 36,000 Pounds

Civilized man has learned to endure extremes of pain, but he has not yet learned how to deal successfully with tension. He drinks although he knows this will cause deterioration of mind and body; he smokes although he has been told that smoking may cause cancer of the lungs and other diseases; he overeats although he knows that heart difficulties, diabetes, and other diseases are augmented by obesity.

Day to day nervousnesses and emotional tension are most easily relieved by habitual eating. The only way to eat habitually without gaining weight is to eat proteins and fats which are inherent in meat. Sugars (carbohydrates) soon cause overweight because they cannot be properly utilized by the human body and are converted into unnecessary body fat.

The lumberjack mentioned earlier eats his beefsteak and is satisfied. Our housewife beset with quibbly problems eats the same dinner and is hungry.

ABNORMAL

HUNGER

CHAPTER SIX

ONE DAY, IN A LITTLE RESTAURANT IN KEMAH, THERE was a vision-lesson for dieters. A 500-pound woman, seated on two chairs, was eating. She was literally shovelling food into her mouth much as coal is shovelled into a coal bin. Both arms were in continuous motion. When one hand put oysters into her mouth, the other hand was picking up a new supply. While it put oysters into her mouth, the other hand reached out for more oysters. When the platter was empty, it was immediately replaced by a platter of fried shrimp, and the arm motions continued without pause. That platter was replaced with fried chicken without causing a pause in the motions. Other diners finished their dinners and reluctantly left without seeing the end of the fat lady's dinner.

This woman obviously had an abnormal hunger. It can be said without exception that when a person consumes quantities of food grossly beyond his body's energy needs, the causes are non-nutritional; they are psychological. People normally eat in excess of their bodily needs for pleasure and for the relief of tensions, but behavior like that described above indicates severe mental illness.

Psychiatrists tell us that some persons regard their huge bodies as fortresses against an unfriendly world. Obesity, especially in adolescence, may be a symbol of rebellious self-reliance and of power. Obesity has been found to represent to some women the desire for pregnancy. On the other hand, obesity is sometimes the method used to escape from admirers who would put in question their femininity. Obesity in some brings about passivity such that the individual avoids the risk of competition in everyday living.

Some persons who overeat do so to gain reassurance on the basis that to be loved is to be fed; in infancy the

Abnormal Hunger

child is fed, and to be fed may later be identified with being loved by husband, by wife, by relative, by friend, or even by the world.

Overeating in normal persons may result from unresolved emotional tensions; it may be the substitute for lack of other gratifications, such as sexual fulfillment, ego-recognition, or achievement. But abnormal overeating or extreme obesity is a symptom of severe emotional illness or psychosis. Finally, abnormal overeating may indicate a true addiction to food. Such individuals, who cannot be weighed on any doctor's scales, obviously require psychiatric help.

There are obvious relations between cultures and food such as the Roman Catholic rejection of meat on Friday, the Orthodox Jewish rituals concerning food, and the Hindu rejection of meat, for example. There are less obvious symbolic meanings, however, which must be recognized if one is to diet successfully. Systematic studies of the symbolic meanings of foods have made possible the following classifications:

Security foods are those eaten in large quantities during periods of stress. Milk, for example, which recalls the dependence of the infant, may be drunk in large quantities when an individual feels the need for emotional security. Refugee children during the war gorged themselves with food, especially with milk, while they felt insecure in their foster homes. When they became more sure of their acceptance and safety, they ceased their frantic eating. If, for any reason, they felt insecure again, they resumed overeating.

Reward foods are those consumed during periods of frustration, when an individual may feel neglected or unappreciated. He may indulge himself with sweets or with special foods to compensate himself for feelings of isolation or unhappiness.

The emotional meanings of foods explain the stress involved in most dieting regimes. When recognized, these emotional supports can sometimes be replaced, enabling the person to diet successfully and to maintain healthful eating habits.

A
MAGIC
WAY

CHAPTER SEVEN

THERE IS A WAY, ALMOST MAGICAL, BY WHICH OBESE INdividuals can quickly reduce from one to two pounds a day. This method consists in the administering of daily shots of one of the natural body hormones, accompanied by a 500-calorie diet which is possible because the hormone enables the person to utilize 2,000 calories a day of his own excess body fat.

This hormone is derived from the urine of pregnant women and has been made commercially available. The substance has the remarkable property of adjusting the systems of both men and women in such a way that excess fat melts away with no discomfort while the patients live on a diet as low as 500 calories a day. Furthermore, the sudden weight loss is not debilitating, nor does it leave the patient with a haggard or drawn look, for only the excess fat is used up.

No additional vitamins are needed in the diet, for no protein foods or vitamins are broken down. The body derives its energy strictly from the excess fat. This treatment has been used successfully with fat diabetics, heart patients, and others to whom it was a great advantage to lose weight quickly.

In all cases including persons of normal health there has been an improvement in general health. Following the administration of this treatment, after a short rest period the treatments can be administered again until the obese person reaches a normal weight. During the interval, patients follow the meat diet. Following the treatment, the desire for excessive amounts of food which seems to characterize some obese persons, appears to be lessened, and such persons can often successfully remain on the meat or modified meat diet.

A Magic Way

Naturally, such a treatment can be administered only by a qualified and interested physician.

Obviously such treatments make no sense unless the person, following the treatment, is determined to maintain his weight loss by a real change in his eating habits. The advantage of the meat diet over the many starvation diets is not merely that it is a more healthful way to reduce; it is a diet which provides plenty of satisfying food for a lifetime.

OVERWEIGHT AND DISEASE

CHAPTER EIGHT

GRAY CLOUD, AN OLD AND WRINKLED INDIAN, SAT BEFORE the fire, drawing a geometrical design with a stick in the dirt before him. Beside him, trying to double their long legs into comfortable positions, sat several visitors from the physiology department of a western university. Gray Cloud was more than 100 years old and had never been sick. No member of his family had ever been sick. Members of his tribe were sick so seldom that the fine new government hospital on the reservation stood unused, and the eager young government doctors fumed at the lack of "business" for them to do.

The visitors were there to discover what was responsible for Gray Cloud's longevity, and what conditions had made the tribe so unnaturally healthy. The college investigators lived with the tribe for several months. They learned how the Indians lived, and what they ate. What they ate was meat! Raw meat, stale meat, sometimes decaying meat, but always meat. In other words the habits of this tribe differed not at all from the habits of other Indians.

The investigators returned to their laboratories to make extensive studies of the effects of a meat and fat diet on the body.

The Indian was a meat eater. He hunted for his food; he did not grow it. He lived in a cave; eventually, he wore a loin cloth and skins for clothing. Today we wear Dior gowns and Ivy League suits. But our stomachs have changed very little.

Many of the serious ailments that beset modern man are made worse by man's getting away from his natural diet, meat, for they are intensified by obesity; in some

Overweight and Disease

cases these diseases are caused by obesity. Some of the diseases definitely related to overweight are: vascular diseases, high blood pressure, coronary occlusions or heart attacks, diabetes, gall bladder diseases, and kidney difficulties.

For every normal-weight person who has a heart attack, there are 10 overweight persons who have heart attacks each year. Diabetes occurs 133 times more frequently in overweight men than it does in normal-weight men and 83 times more frequently in overweight women than it does in normal-weight women. Digestive diseases are 68 percent more frequent in overweight men than in normal-weight men, and vascular diseases are 53 percent more frequent in overweight men than in normal-weight men.

Most overweight diabetics can be relieved of all symptoms and even have their laboratory tests revert to normal if they lose their excess fat. Such patients can remain without symptoms if they keep their weight down and this can best be accomplished by means of the meat diet.

Even thin diabetics benefit from eating large quantities of protein and fat and can build their bodies up to a normal weight by the use of these foods. With thin diabetics, however, medication continues to be required although formerly fat and reduced diabetics can often dispense with insulin entirely.

Fat tissue is a tremendous user of insulin. An overweight diabetic must produce a great quantity of insulin to keep the fat cells living. These divert insulin from its normal activity of supplying the vital organs, such as the heart, brain, lungs, etc., and the insulin is then consumed by the worthless body fat deposited by the eating of incorrect foodstuffs.

Although the entire problem concerning diabetes has not been solved, it seems apparent that such individuals cannot derive adequate energy or utilize properly exogenous (eaten) sugar. Consequently, if large amounts of protein and fat are supplied through food, the diabetic does not break down his own body resources to supply needed energy.

In regard to high blood pressure it can be stated unequivocally that most physicians endeavor to reduce their overweight hypertensive patients as their first step of treatment. Here again, eighteen years of clinical practice has provided convincing proof that there is no meth-

Overweight and Disease

od of weight loss to equal the improvements attained through the eating of meat. Former prejudices against the use of meat as the preferred food in such cases are disappearing because of studies showing that the heart works less in the digestion of meat than of grains and other foods. Meat goes into rapid solution and easy absorption in the intestinal tract.

Light salads, sometimes recommended for summer fare, are much less easily digested than meat. Consequently, the overweight, hypertensive patient should continue his meat diet right on through the hottest summer months.

Many sufferers with gall bladder difficulties have been told at some time not to eat meat, doubtless because of the mistaken idea that meat is hard to digest. If one has a sluggish gall bladder, the eating of fat will stimulate and tend to empty the organ, thereby helping it to function more properly.

Fat is a powerful tonic to the gall bladder. This fact can be vividly seen in gall bladder x-ray procedures where a fatty meal is given to cause the contraction and emptying of the gall bladder. Obviously, individuals consuming meat are less susceptible to gall bladder ailments since the fat in the meat keeps the gall bladder functioning and toned up, thus reducing the likelihood of this organ becoming sluggish and retaining insipid bile leading to infections and deposition of stones.

Excess fat is a great burden to the heart. Unlike dead weight which could be carried on the shoulders, the heart must not only help the body to carry the weight of excess fat, it must pump blood to each of these unnecessary fat cells. This strain on the heart is undoubtedly the greatest contributing factor involved in coronary occlusions (heart attacks). To prevent a heart attack or to treat a person who has had a coronary occlusion, the first necessity is to see that he loses weight.

THE CHOLESTEROL CRAZE

CHAPTER NINE

CHOLESTEROL HAS HAD MORE NOTICES IN THE RECENT press than many a movie star, and some of the discussion about this substance has reflected much misinformation.

Cholesterol, which is to be found in the blood stream and in most foods, has no proved connections with that blocking of the heart arteries known as coronary occlusion. Because the amount of cholesterol in the total blood stream has been found in some patients to be high at the time of a heart attack, a connection of cholesterol with the heart attack has in some cases been assumed, whereas it is a fact that many normal, healthy individuals have an equally high cholesterol content in the blood stream without experiencing heart difficulties of any kind.

Occlusion is the blocking of one or more coronary arteries by a nodule or nodules within the wall of the artery. Within such a nodule have been found deposits of particles of one component of cholesterol, that known as the SF 12-20 fraction. The liver daily manufactures fifteen grams of cholesterol including in this amount some SF 12-20. If foods containing cholesterol are eaten, the liver manufactures less cholesterol. If a diet low in cholesterol is eaten, the liver manufactures more cholesterol, including some of the special fraction called SF 12-20. In other words, the more cholesterol is eaten, the less the liver is stimulated to produce its own cholesterol with its relatively high proportion of SF 12-20.

The ingestion of foods that contain cholesterol such as meat, which contains cholesterol because of its fat content, does not contribute to the development of these nodules or to the deposition of material in them. As a matter of fact, it can be shown that the reverse is true, for protein which is conspicuously found in meat, has a strong tendency to lower the blood cholesterol level.

The Cholesterol Craze

Protein is about the only substance that can produce the lowering of the blood cholesterol.

Furthermore, if one were to limit his diet to foods not containing cholesterol, a diet which would be so unpalatable and contrary to human appetite that it would be almost impossible to eat, the cholesterol level of the blood would increase. In fact, individuals on starvation diets or suffering from malnutrition have an increase in blood cholesterol, and more significantly they also have an increase in SF 12-20 particles. The reason for the increase in this component is that as protein intake goes down, trouble arises in the handling of cholesterol by the body.

A group of diabetic children who were maintained on a low protein diet developed vascular lesions after fifteen years and after twenty-one years very few of them were alive. This mistaken experiment was conducted under the belief that a low protein and/or low cholesterol diet would prevent these complications, whereas in fact it intensified them.

The Indonesians consume much fat and their diet is rich in cholesterol; yet they have a low incidence of coronary disease. The Japanese subsist on a diet containing a minimum of cholesterol and fatty foods; practically no grease is used in their cooking. However, these people have a relatively high disease rate of "heart attacks." It is reasonable to conjecture the possibility that the high incidence of coronary disease in the Japanese is due to their cholesterol-poor diet. Such diets cause the production of more cholesterol by the liver, and this cholesterol may be rich in SF 12-20, the fraction which has been found to occur in the nodules in the coronary.

There is much that is unknown concerning the cause of coronary disease. Men, for example, have such illness ten times more frequently than women, regardless of the diet eaten; also the onset of the disease occurs six to eight years earlier than in women. People deficient in thyroid are more prone to the deposition of nodules in their blood vessels and to coronary disease. Meat is an excellent food for such people for the protein increases the activity of the thyroid. Only two substances have been shown to alter the advance of artery disease, protein and thyroid.

Certain sellers of unsaturated fats and oils, substances which are low in cholesterol, have unduly claimed that by the use of their product and the elimination of animal fat, the progression of coronary disease can be retarded or the disease avoided. These claims are not justified. Indeed the food and drug administration have warned the sellers to refrain from making such unjustified claims. Most experts do not believe that the adding of a vegetable or unsaturated oil to the diet will lower the cholesterol content of the blood or alleviate artery diseases.

Eskimos eat a tremendous amount of meat and fat. When an Eskimo child thinks of a treat while visiting the local trading post, he thinks of a piece of fat. Yet the incidence of coronary disease and even of high blood pressure in Eskimos is quite low. Although animal fat contains cholesterol, investigators have shown that there is no correlation between the total blood cholesterol and the tendency to develop vascular disease.

A group of subjects was given a diet containing an enormous amount of fat—so great in fact that the fat had to be melted and eaten with a spoon. Yet these subjects developed no ill effects and no signs of vascular difficulties. They thrived upon their diet.

In one of Chicago's largest medical centers, a group of critically ill people, who were in terminal stages of cancer and had to be fed through tubes, were found to be wasting away with the usual tube feeding. Consequently, large amounts of fat were melted and fed these patients. It was soon noted that the patients gained weight and that their general condition improved.

The real enemy of the heart is not cholesterol but excess body fat. During World War II it was noted that American soldiers 35 years and younger had a relatively high number of coronary diseases whereas British soldiers of the same age group, genetically alike, who smoked alike, were trained alike, had a much lower incidence. The big difference between the two armies was the food eaten. The large amount of carbohydrates in the form of candy, cake, chewing gum, and soda pop in the diet of the Americans caused excess weight, and added poundage is the biggest factor in the development of coronary disease.

It was also learned during World War II that when the Germans moved into Oslo and food became scarce, the incidence of coronary occlusion dropped amazingly. After the war when the amount of food rose to pre-war levels and weight increased, the incidence of heart attacks increased rapidly.

Overweight leads to a high degree of vascular disease and death from it. Greater longevity and freedom from such disease is found among those who are normal in weight.

YOUR BEST FRIENDS ARE YOUR WORST ENEMIES

CHAPTER TEN

HOSPITALITY CAN WRECK ALMOST ANY DIET IF THE DIETER is not careful. How can one refuse that homemade dessert that the den mothers have made for the boy scout meeting? In fact, how can one refuse any one of two or three desserts? The best way is to accept a piece of that wonderful cake, take fork in hand and LOOK as if you are eating. Drink your coffee instead. If you wield your fork correctly, without taking a single bite, you can deceive the most hospitable hostess.

How I Lost 36,000 Pounds

There is something about dieting that is a challenge to all your friends—a challenge to them to make you forget your diet. It is usually best to tell no one that you are dieting. Actually the meat diet is not a diet; it is a change in eating habits that needs no explaining.

Friends want you to be like them; most of them are overweight, and they are envious of anyone who has the self-discipline to restrict his eating habits for health or other reasons.

Visits, to a restaurant or to a friend's house for a meal, should be dealt with in the same way. Every restaurant and almost every host serves meat of some kind. Nearly every host serves potatoes. Eat what your diet calls for, but accept servings of other things, and no one will notice that you do not eat them. At a restaurant, order what you can eat unless your host orders for you; then do as suggested above.

If you are tempted by friendship to forget your diet and "go along" with your friends, remember the preceeding week and how you have disciplined yourself. If you eat what is not on your diet, the resulting pleasure lasts but a few minutes, whereas your weight loss, if you stick to it, can be permanent. Your friends will admire

Your Best Friends Are Your Worst Enemies

you more when you are thinner, even if you resist their invitations in order to get that way. Going out is no excuse for nibbling the forbidden which will render useless all your earlier self-denial.

The inner struggle between one's desire to weigh the right amount and the desire to satisfy psychological or physical cravings is difficult enough. It is intensified many times, however, by the pressure of family and friends who sometimes act like the devil's advocates in their hospitable efforts to break down your disciplined eating.

Teenagers or younger children who are overweight are especially susceptible to the suggestions of their peers. Perhaps they can gain the respect of their friends who want to stop at the hamburger bar by ordering a grown-up cup of coffee or tea instead of by ordering that fattening hamburger. They must remind themselves of the coming encounter with the scales.

EATING

FOR

BEAUTY

CHAPTER ELEVEN

BEAUTY IS A WORD WITH MANY DEFINITIONS. WHEN IT is applied to the human body, it has as many definitions as there are cultures. Reflect, for example, upon the differences between a buxom German beauty and a delicate Japanese charmer. Each is handsome by the standards of her own country but not a beauty in the eyes of the other's countrymen.

Even within a single culture, the Western-European culture for example, there are almost as many definitions of a beautiful woman as there are countries. Some of these visions of beauty differ from the American ideal.

The beauty of woman may depend upon her conformity to an ideal type as to skin color, hair color and texture, body shape, and weight. Even distribution of weight may be a factor in evaluating a woman's beauty. In Syria for example, large hips and heavy thighs are greatly admired in a marriageable female. In the France of fifty years ago, fullness about the neck, shoulders and arms was considered desirable, although today French ideals of beauty of form are more like the slender ideal American beauty.

America's ideal of today is similar to that of ancient Rome where mothers are said to have starved their daughters to make them appear more desirable as marriage partners. The American ideal of today is the opposite of that of ancient Tunisia where women were put in restricted quarters and discouraged from exercise while they were fed all manner of delicious food to fatten them before marriage.

Indeed, today, the average middle-aged American, man or woman, suffers a double tragedy, for he departs both from the American ideal of beauty and from that

Eating for Beauty

of health. In America, from 20 to 40 percent of those examined for life-insurance are from 10 to 20 percent overweight. In fact, statistics gathered from diverse sources reveal such a high incidence of obesity in the adult American population that overweight is called the most frequent physical abnormality and has become a pressing medical problem.

Furthermore, when a person is more than 10 percent overweight, his excess weight tends to increase with age, making him more and more obese in the middle age and in later years when obesity becomes truly a health hazard because of the strain it puts upon the heart and other organs.

Some tables of ideal or average height and weight correspondences have in the past failed to take into account differences in frame or bone structure. The tables here given are newly compiled and represent the latest and best medical and statistical conclusions of advantageous height and weight correspondence from the point of view of health. Fortunately, the ideal of health bears a close resemblance to the ideal American shape which emphasizes slenderness with "bones showing" so to speak.

How I Lost 36,000 Pounds

Even though the middle-aged American tends toward the beginnings of obesity, he is by no means resigned to it as is evidenced by his maintenance of slenderness as an ideal. In fact, obesity has come to be synonymous with laziness, slowness of thought and action, and other unattractive characteristics. Even that comic character, the happy fat man, has changed; he has become the sad fat man. Since a fat man is never taken very seriously, he is even funnier when he is sad. And it is a truism to point out that every fat person is sad. He eats because he is sad. And he is sad because he eats—a horrible circle which he can break out of if he will, for on the meat diet he can both eat and get thin.

WEIGHT CHARTS

CHAPTER TWELVE

EACH INDIVIDUAL HAS A WEIGHT THAT IS RIGHT FOR HIS body and no chart can accurately designate that weight. Only his own body, after months of eating the proper foods, can tell him what his weight should be. An approximation, however, may be helpful, and the following chart based on body-build and pressure studies by the Metropolitan Life Insurance Company is probably the most accurate available. (Ordinary charts of average weight have been calculated on a basis of the population-at-large. Since this includes the overweight segment, weights considered "average" pertain to those of an overweight population, and such weights are considerably higher than "desirable" weights.)

Studies emphasize that persons' "normal" body weight exhibit differences in their fatness; body weight is an imperfect guide to body fat.

Weight in Pounds According to Frame (In Indoor Clothing)

DESIRABLE WEIGHTS FOR MEN of ages 25 and over

HEIGHT (with shoes on) 1-inch heels Feet / Inches	SMALL FRAME	MEDIUM FRAME	LARGE FRAME
5 2	112–120	118–129	126–141
5 3	115–123	121–133	129–144
5 4	118–126	124–136	132–148
5 5	121–129	127–139	135–152
5 6	124–133	130–143	138–156
5 7	128–137	134–147	142–161
5 8	132–141	138–152	147–166
5 9	136–145	142–156	151–170
5 10	140–150	146–160	155–174
5 11	144–154	150–165	159–179
6 0	148–158	154–170	164–184
6 1	152–162	158–175	168–189
6 2	156–167	162–180	173–194
6 3	160–171	167–185	178–199
6 4	164–175	172–190	182–204

DESIRABLE WEIGHTS FOR WOMEN of ages 25 and over

HEIGHT (with shoes on) 2-inch heels Feet / Inches	SMALL FRAME	MEDIUM FRAME	LARGE FRAME
4 10	92– 98	96–107	104–119
4 11	94–101	98–110	106–122
5 0	96–104	101–113	109–125
5 1	99–107	104–116	112–128
5 2	102–110	107–119	115–131
5 3	105–113	110–122	118–134
5 4	108–116	113–126	121–138
5 5	111–119	116–130	125–142
5 6	114–123	120–135	129–146
5 7	118–127	124–139	133–150
5 8	122–131	128–143	137–154
5 9	126–135	132–147	141–158
5 10	130–140	136–151	145–163
5 11	134–144	140–155	149–168
6 0	138–148	144–159	153–173

For girls between 18 and 25, subtract 1 pound for each year under 25.

*This table was prepared by Metropolitan Life Insurance Co.

OBESITY

IN

CHILDREN

CHAPTER THIRTEEN

PARENTS SHOULD BE EDUCATED TO PREVENT OBESITY IN children. Overweight children become overweight adults. Since an increasing number of juveniles are growing fat, it can be said that we are eating our way to the cemetery beginning in infancy.

There is a widespread impression among parents that to be big is to be strong and healthy. As a result, children are given an excessive amount of food. It may be true that among animals the larger ones have more prowess than the smaller, but this largeness is not fat; it is inherent body structure. Fortunately, in man, size is not the criterion for importance. Actually, excess fat makes an individual less, not more, physically and mentally able. The habit of overeating is acquired, not inherited.

The child's birth weight bears no relationship to subsequent obesity. Most overweight children studied have one or both parents overweight. Then how can it be true that obesity is not inherited? It can be shown that an overweight parent constantly urges his or her child to overeat or constantly sets an example of over-eating; that in the family eating a great deal is associated with well-being or happiness.

Obesity in many children starts within two years of age, in others after four years of age. Glandular disease is rarely found to be the cause of obesity in children, and faulty glands should not even be suspected unless the child's height is below normal.

Obesity is just as harmful to children as it is to grown persons. An infant weighing 20 pounds, whose normal weight is 15 pounds, is in the same situation as his father, who weighs 225 pounds when he should weigh

Obesity in Children

175. Because a youth's vital organs are newer and more toned, they can carry excess fat easier than they can later in life; nevertheless, the strain weakens the organs and contributes to possible malfunctioning. In any person, even though he is young, obesity causes lethargy, fatigue, and shortness of breath. Furthermore, life insurance companies have shown that overweight infants do not live as long as the less well-fed babies. Actual deprivation of food is less of a health hazard for a baby than overfeeding.

The problem of obesity in young adults has its roots in their infancy. Mothers are convinced that their babies are healthier if they are plump or fat. Indeed it may be that a chubby little cherub is a cuddly, irresistible darling who outwardly disarms us and whose cheeks we feel inclined to pinch, but actually such an adorable baby has a heart, lungs, and kidneys functioning overtime because of that excess weight. Furthermore, one rarely finds an overweight infant or child who is not also anemic. In addition, the digestive tracts of such children are overloaded and working to capacity thus inclining them to colic and to other intestinal problems.

Once habits of improper eating are established in children, the resultant obesity is nearly impossible to correct. Years of eating-conditioning fostered on a child by loved ones cannot be eradicated by the advice of a physician or even by "average" personal motivation. What is required is a resolute act of the will. Threats, pressures from society, and even ridicule do not correct obesity in the young, for food is too closely related to comfort and to the love from parents. Besides, the desire to emulate a loved, heavy mother or father may be great. The parent may think that the child will just "grow out of it," but it is not so. What is required is a decision on the part of the child, and sometimes on the part of the parent, if the child is very young; in addition there is required on the part of the young person a resolute act of the will. If the parents and the brothers and sisters are thin, there is a better chance that overweight in a particular child will regress after puberty.

It is practically impossible to effect obesity in children under ten; the problem in adolescents is about as difficult. Adolescents are impervious to arguments that obesity is injurious to health and will affect their longevity, for they are inclined to feel omnipotent with an eternity of life before them. But some adolescents are motivated to lose weight in order to gain popularity or to excel in sports, or to eliminate acne. (And it may be said here that food does not cause or effect acne. Neither sugars nor fats in the diet affect it in any way.)

Many young persons lose weight for a week or more in order to wear a particular dress or to look thinner for a particular occasion such as the school prom, but once the specific need is attained they revert to old eating habits. Fad diets, consequently, are valueless for permanent results; at the first minor frustration or need for attention, old eating habits are re-established.

Parents should cease rewarding children for eating. If a child is conditioned to feel that by poking additional food into his system he pleases and conciliates his parents, later in life he will have learned these responses as surely as did Pavlov's dogs.

WHAT ABOUT MILK?

CHAPTER FOURTEEN

ANIMALS, EXCEPT FOR MAN, WEAN THEIR BABIES FROM milk as soon as the young can obtain the type of food eaten by the adult. The time of this weaning varies from as little as a few days for the baby agouti (a South American rodent), who starts to nibble leaves within an hour after birth, to months as in the case of cattle.

Man apparently decided that if milk was good for growing infants, it should be good for all stages of his life. Faith in the food value of milk is especially prevalent in the United States, although some ethnic groups in this country, and many in other countries do not share the strong tradition of milk drinking to be found here.

Because of this strong tradition, although a baby normally begins to refuse milk at about seven months, his parents often insist upon giving it to him. The more the infant resists, the more the parents insist, since they are convinced that their child will not develop as well without this food. Their determination forces the child to accept milk, and this conditioning of the child continues throughout his life.

In many cases rewards are provided for the child who drinks all of the milk served him. On reaching adulthood, consequently, most individuals are convinced that milk is "the food" and any facts to the contrary are considered to be anti-God, anti-home, and anti-country.

Like adults, babies fed large amounts of milk become quite heavy from excess fat tissue, but also like adults on a similar diet, they lack muscle development and are often deficient in blood iron resulting in iron deficiency anemia. When infants are fed large amounts of milk, protein foods such as meat, fish, fowl, and eggs are not

What about Milk?

eaten, and lack of these foods results in important deficiencies in bodily development.

Pre-school children who are milk drinkers usually consume excessive amounts of starchy foods and sweets, which they conveniently wash down with more milk.

Aside from the excess weight resulting from the excessive use of milk, anemia is one of the major disorders associated with its use. Iron substances will not dissolve in milk; milk, consequently, is "iron poor." Furthermore, if iron is added to milk it will precipitate. In other words, not only is milk deficient in the iron needed to develop rich blood, but if other foods containing this element are eaten when milk is present in the intestinal tract, the iron in these other foods is precipitated and not made available to the blood. Thus a severe iron-deficiency anemia may result. Recently, some of the manufacturers of milk for infant feeding have recognized this problem of milk anemia and have found ways of adding iron to their product. They still do not acknowledge, however, that the milk itself constitutes the problem.

These anemias do not occur, however, in infants with a diet rich in solid, protein foods. Experience indicates that the most dramatically strong and healthy infants are those who were given milk for only two or three months and then given solid, protein foods.

During my earlier years as a general practitioner, I followed the teaching of my school in prescribing a quart of milk a day for expectant mothers. This I did especially rigorously because many of my patients had not been conscious of their dental needs and had poor teeth, and I had been trained to believe that milk provided the needed calcium for bones and teeth.

I never questioned the role of milk when I noticed that my pregnant patients who followed instructions lost their teeth more rapidly than those who did not drink the prescribed milk. Medical findings revealed the reason, however. Indeed there is a high concentration of calcium in milk, but this calcium is bound to other substances in the milk, and in this bound-up form the milk calcium cannot pass through the intestinal wall into the blood stream. Furthermore, foods containing calcium in a form available to the blood, when eaten with milk, are divested of the calcium by the milk so that they too cannot supply the needed calcium in a form that can pass through the intestinal wall.

In fact, the drinking of excessive quantities of milk actually causes a deficiency of blood calcium. Kidney

What about Milk?

stones are sometimes found in heavy milk drinkers, probably the result of the effort of the body's chemical laboratory to remove calcium from the bones and teeth in order to correct this deficiency.

In addition to the other misconceptions about milk already mentioned, the benefits attributed to milk drinking in the case of ulcer patients can be shown erroneous. Treatment of such patients with milk is now obsolete. The basis for using a milk diet in such cases was the fact that milk is an anti-acid and as such neutralized the excess acid in the stomach. Although this is the case, it has been noted that once the acid in the stomach is neutralized, a rebound phenomena occurs in approximately one-half hour such that the stomach reacts to the milk and more acid is formed so that the degree of acidity is greater than that before the milk was ingested.

The ulcer patient now has additional discomfort, and if he is unaware of what is happening, he may drink more milk and repeat the cycle. In addition such an ulcer patient may gain weight due to the milk and become more susceptible to heart trouble.

Other conditions, such as ulcerative colitis, once believed to be alleviated by a bland milk diet, have been shown to be lessened following the removal of milk from the patient's diet.

Although some believe that these ill effects result from allergy to milk, it is my belief that they result because milk is basically intolerable to any mammal after infancy.

THE
HUNGRY
ANONYMOUS

CHAPTER FIFTEEN

IT HAS ALREADY BEEN NOTED THAT OVEREATING IS OFTEN a way of lessening tensions or of substituting for satisfactions that are missing from the overweight person's life. These facts were constructively utilized in certain experiments in Boston where a social club of obese persons, similar in some respects to Alcoholics Anonymous, was formed. A group of individuals who found themselves unable to lose by the usual methods, but who were sincerely determined to reduce, met together with the consent of their physicians and formed a social club.

How I Lost 36,000 Pounds

The purpose of the club was mutual encouragement, and it was found that overweight persons meeting together once a week can effectively encourage each other to maintain regular weight loss. The experimental group met once a week for sixteen weeks for stimulating discussion of their mutual problem and of general nutritional principles. Members of the group discovered that as they received satisfaction from communicating their problems and from sharing the problems of others, their desire for food decreased.

In fact, so successful was this project during the experimental stage that informal meetings of the members continued after the formal experiment was over. Weight loss continued, and the members expressed the conviction that a significant method had been devised to assist them with their problems.

If the patient receives satisfaction from other persons through companionship and appreciation of others for the powerful inner drives to eat, then the need to ingest food diminishes. This explains why obesity may be decreased by means of the formation of social clubs similar to Alcoholics Anonymous. Such clubs formed throughout the nation might prove to be an important factor in dealing with the national problem of obesity.

LIFE WITHOUT FOOD

CHAPTER SIXTEEN

SOME LIVES ARE NOT WORTH LIVING WITHOUT FOOD. To an individual who looks forward more to deep-dish apple pie than he does to anything else he can think of, life would not be worth living without that pie or its equivalent of some rich, succulent dish. A forty-five-year-old man seeking treatment for hypertension, may decide, subconsciously or consciously, that he would rather eat than be handsome, or healthy.

A sixty-eight-year-old man, even one who has suffered one coronary occlusion, may decide that his life is empty without the rich desserts he looked forward to.

A human being has the right to make such decisions, and no persuasions by family or physicians can dissuade a man from eating if he has made up his mind that his life's happiness depends upon food. Some persons can be re-educated to find satisfactions in other ways, and thus can be, so to speak, weaned from their faulty food habits. Others resist this retraining, and for those no diet will work, for they will not follow any diet that deprives them of their loved and satisfying foods. The most earnest physician is forced to admit failure in such cases. Indeed, once he recognizes that he is encountering such a food-addict, he may even ask himself if he has the right to remove a human being's one remaining pleasure—the one thing that makes living worth while.

It is for the remainder of the population that this book is written. It is written for all those who have long been struggling with their overweight, who have been disappointed in the food-fad starvation diets, or for those who have been struggling in vain with their own appetites. It advocates a re-education of the person and what is actually a refreshment of the body without starvation and without the fatigue that a starvation diet causes. Furthermore, it advocates a sensible diet that is actually not a diet at all, but is rather a re-examination of eating habits. It says: Eat meat and grow thin, and it is based on eighteen years of experience in the general practice of medicine.

MODIFICATION OF THE MEAT DIET

CHAPTER SEVENTEEN

THIS DIET IS A SUSTAINING ONE, NOT A REDUCING DIET and should not be resorted to until a dietary plateau has been reached on the meat diet, until, in other words, no weight has been lost for two weeks on the meat diet. Most people who begin the modified diet after losing satisfactorily with the first diet find that their weight increases about five pounds, but that it is then maintained there. The new diet must be followed as religiously as the old one in order to maintain the new weight.

MODIFIED MEAT DIET

EAT ALL YOU WANT OF

    Meat

    Fish

    Fowl

    Eggs

    Natural Cheese (processed cheese is prepared with sugar)

    These foods may be broiled, baked, or fried, without batter, meal or flour.

EAT A LIMITED AMOUNT OF

    1 vegetable (preferably one that is listed on the meat diet)

    and

    1 fruit (preferably one listed on the meat diet)

    Use small to moderate portions, about equal to an ice-cream scoopful.

DRINK ALL YOU WANT OF

    Coffee

    Tea

    Water

    and nothing else.

DEAR DOCTOR

CHAPTER EIGHTEEN

THE PROBLEM OF OBESITY HAS INVOLVED A SMALL segment of my interest in the practice of general medicine and surgery; however, overweight patients are ubiquitous and come to every physician's attention. Many consulting the doctor for other matters have excess fat that requires losing before health is attained.

Colleagues have asked me the reason for my better-than-average success in treating obesity. The meat diet described in this book is infallible if followed. I am convinced that it is the only correct way to lose poundage. It is physiological and natural to man. The elimination of sugars, breads and other foods not inherent to man's need will effect some weight loss, but attaining a normal weight and developing a real change in eating habits require the meat diet.

In exceedingly obese cases or where rapid loss is desirable, chorionic gonadotropic hormone along with a 500 calorie diet is given. The method has been effective and safe. The technique consists of giving subcutaneously 500 International Units of the hormone every day for a total of 21 injections. Sundays may be missed. The 500 calorie diet is as follows:

> Eat only 2 meals a day (breakfast-supper, supper-lunch, or any other combination). Each meal consists of all of the following:
>
> 1/5 lb. lean meat
> 1 Zwieback
> 1 serving (1/2 cup) of low calorie vegetable
> 1 small apple or orange
> tablespoon milk in 24 hours
> juice of 1 lemon in 24 hours
> coffee, tea, water—ad. lib.
> salt and pepper—ad. lib.

Dear Doctor

No deviation, addition or omission, must occur. Two pounds are lost daily. The hormone allows the body to derive 2000 calories a day from excess fat. The 500 exogenous calories and the former 2000 provide a total of 2500 calories.

Some patients feel "full" and eat less than the stipulated diet, later excusing themselves for eating bits of other foods. It is important to eat all the food listed for maximum weight loss. Since there is residual hormone in the body, the 500 calorie diet may be continued for three days after the injections are finished. A loss of one pound a day is satisfactory, but two pounds is much better. The weight loss is not deleterious, but healthful. The meat diet is started or resumed after the injections to effect additional weight loss and correct eating habits.

Additional courses of the hormone can be given. Each course is preceded by intervals of at least six weeks on the meat diet. The manufacturers of the medicine advise as to possible intolerances and reactions. In the several hundred patients I have treated to date, none have occurred.

The above methods provide excellent approaches to the problem of obesity, but this is not the total answer.

The psychology of the patient is the variable, not the diets. Emotional factors may make impossible the changing of oral pleasures.

The physician needs to have much determination in helping the overweight. He has to provide constant encouragement, empathy and authority for the patient. Disappointments in patients' cooperation and resultant frustrations are the rule. Stamina is required. Rewards for these dogged efforts should produce permanently normal weights in two out of five patients.

SOME

MUST

REMAIN FAT

CHAPTER NINETEEN

IT IS POSSIBLE TO ELIMINATE THE PROBLEM OF OBESITY in the human race. All that is required is the exclusive use of protein and fat and the abolishment of carbohydrate. Carbohydrate causes fat to be deposited and, also, prevents this fat from being utilized. These effects vary in degree in individuals. Some are less prone than others to the influence of carbohydrate. For example, members of the same family, eating the same food may vary in their amounts of body fat. Yet, carbohydrates create and store excess adipose tissue in everyone, even thin people.

How I Lost 36,000 Pounds

Slender persons are quite aware of a few pounds weight gain causing an unpleasant tightness in their clothes. Nevertheless, civilized man has accepted carbohydrate-type foods so completely, and made them such an integral part of his life that it is impossible to avoid their use. The use of carbohydrate is impregnated in our civilization and cannot be avoided any more than drinking or smoking, regardless of the health factors involved. Thus, in some degree all must remain fat.

In the markedly overweight, the problem is more complicated and not simply related to culture and heritage. Profound subconscious and conscious reasons are involved. Obesity is an adjustment to emotional conditions that would otherwise be intolerable. These factors must be considered and rectified for they obviate any method used to reduce; furthermore, curtailing excessive eating and interfering with this adjustment might cause more serious maladjustment.

Although suicide is a gloomy theme, and people avoid the subject, it is necessary to consider the subject as it pertains to obesity.

Freud postulated that there is in many people a death instinct, which only rarely causes one to actually commit suicide. Psychiatrists have confirmed this finding. As one matures, this destructive instinct is restrained by directing its force outward to other objects; it is further opposed by life instincts (love) that produce a constructive personality. In some, the personality fails to develop adequately, and the instinct to destroy oneself remains. Some kill themselves quickly, or slowly, or not at all or postpone death by making concessions. Eating resulting in marked obesity and poor health is a form of concession—the price paid for living. Obese people rarely are consciously aware of the bargaining. They blame their obesity on fate, glands, heredity, physical defects, and joy of eating. They do not accept the responsibility of their self-destruction. My own experience with the obese shows that their instinct toward self-destruction is highly developed, as the following examples illustrate.

Mr. C. R. G. had a severe "heart attack." He was 61, 5' 7" tall and weighed 192 pounds. After a slow and difficult recovery he was discharged from the hospital and given the "meat diet" to attain a normal weight. Six weeks of successful dieting resulted in his losing twelve pounds. He failed to keep subsequent office appointments and I did not see him again until many months later. At that time I was called to see Mr. G. because he was having another severe "heart attack." His wife told me

How I Lost 36,000 Pounds

that her husband had failed to return for the scheduled follow-up visits because he didn't want to stay on a diet. If Mr. G. had continued to diet and lose weight, he probably would be alive today.

* * *

Mrs. M. S. F. has six children; her religious convictions obviate her avoiding further pregnancy. Consequently, she and her husband have agreed to refrain from marital relations. The family is semi-indigent and they are constantly in debt. Mrs. F. doesn't go anywhere or participate in outside recreational activity; for aside from money problems the husband enjoys staying home watching television, and her elderly mother, who lives in the home, insists that a "mother's place is in the home" taking care of the children. The mother scolds even if she leaves the children to attend church alone. About the only escape Mrs. F. has from boredom is through visits to free clinics where she seeks a cure for her obesity.

She is 35 years of age, 5' 6" and weighs 233 pounds. No one has been able to help her lose; in fact, her size is in a constant uptrend.

Recently, Mrs. F. has been referred to a psychiatrist who learned that subconsciously Mrs. F. wished to attack

Some Must Remain Fat

and destroy her family. The mother, husband and children thwart and deprive her need for personal satisfactions and comforts. Demands of the family bring forth strong, aggressive feelings which she restrains because of a highly developed conscience, fear of retaliation and love. Her hatred is incompletely neutralized and is turned within herself; in addition, the malice creates guilt feelings demanding that she be punished.

Mrs. F.'s instinctive wish to die is augmented by an unhappy and despoiled existence. Obesity allows her wish to make a subconscious compromise. She manages to punish and avenge herself by excessive eating. Her weight prevents keeping up with routine housework and requires the 68-year-old mother do a goodly share. Her husband is kept in a state of anxiety because he fears for her health and his interest in her diet and treatments affords her much attention. The children are cared for, but are made aware of the great physical effort required to provide this solicitousness.

If a way were found to reduce Mrs. F., she would be deprived of a method for handling her insufferable existence. Her aggressive and guilt feeling would be overwhelming and her attenuated suicide might be replaced by a more rapid form of self-destruction. Overeating shortens life, but it takes longer for the heart, brain and other vital organs to succumb to fat than to more potent poisons. The entire problem is complicated by the ebullition of pleasure in the act of eating. Delight in this erotic torture adds to its continuation. Further, Mrs. F.'s maladjustment is augmented by friends and relatives who criticize her obesity, but ply her with food.

Instead of body growth, self-love and self-hate, Mrs. F. needs a personality growth, investment of love in the outside world and direction of hatred upon proper objects.

* * *

Mrs. A. Y. is a highly intelligent, educated middle-aged widow. An unhappy marriage ended when her husband succumbed to the effects of alcohol. After several years of loneliness, she met a man with whom a love affair developed. The affair lasted over a year, and was terminated suddenly when Mrs. Y. received a letter from him saying he had left the city and did not wish to see her again.

Mrs. Y. developed an immediate, severe melancholy which worsened progressively. One day her son found her in an alcoholic stupor and she was admitted to the hospital. In the hospital, she neglected herself completely, even refusing to use the toilet facilities. Psychiatric treatment helped, but real improvement occurred simultaneously with her interest in food. Her appetite became voracious. The more she ate, and the fatter she became, the more her spirits rose. Her usual weight was 108 pounds, but on leaving the hospital she scaled 146 pounds despite her 5' 2".

Psychiatric studies revealed that Mrs. Y.'s eating was her mode of adjusting to an intolerable life situation. It was a form of self-destruction, but a substitute for suicide. Fantasies and dreams divulged the patient's desire to commit murder—to murder her lover and herself. She had intense resentment to the interruption of her invested love. This love had helped neutralize her instinctive, destructive feelings and now these were unbridled. Fear of retaliation by society and persistent love for this man inhibited her killing him; instead, the destructive impulses were directed back upon herself.

It is known that in the infantile areas of the mind, one may behave as though the body of someone else is included in one's own. This phantasy is called "introjection" because a particular person seems to be brought into the self. One may say, for example, he carries his love for someone inside himself.

In the primitive, mental process these terms are not symbolic but factual. Mrs. Y. introjected her sweetheart; excessive eating and weight gain helped make the adoption more real for Mrs. Y. The immature personality retains its childlike associations of oral gratification, and such people express their love with their mouths, much as a suckling infant. This type of individual cannot stand being denied and when Mrs. Y.'s lover abandoned her, she hated him intensively because of the deprivation. She felt hopeless, as though she would die. The act of eating—biting—is one mixed with love and hate. The nursing child consumes the milk of the mother avidly, but if she denies the child and removes the nipple, his sucking efforts increase to such a degree that he tries to consume not only milk but the breast as well. Eating is a form of devouring. During certain ceremonies, some religions practice the eating and drinking of food which is supposed to symbolize the taking into oneself the body and blood of the loved leader. Eating symbolized for Mrs. Y. the oral incorporation of her lover and at the same time satisfied her infantile need for love. Her hate and aggressiveness produced feelings of extreme guilt. She felt the need to be punished to make atonement. The humiliation and the physical handicaps resulting from obesity were her reconciliations. Also, excessive gain in weight was a blow against the gentleman, too, for he always admired her slim figure. Thus, in many ways Mrs. Y.'s excessive eating helped her relieve an intolerable situation within the conformity of her incomplete personality. To remove the assuaging power of food would cause Mrs. Y. despair and unbearable suffering; nevertheless, she is now seeking a doctor to give her a diet and some pills to reduce.

Marked obesity then involves the total personality—mentally, emotionally and physically—and the problem cannot have a simple solution.

CASES

MRS. R. J. E., A FORTY-SEVEN-YEAR-OLD WHITE FEMALE, came to the office complaining that she had a weight problem. She weighed 230 and one-half pounds. She had two children and had been married twenty-three years. Prior to her marriage, her weight was relatively normal for her age and height, but after her marriage she began to gain, and her weight had been abnormal for much of that time. A physical examination, including an examination of the thyroid, revealed that her organs were normal and functioning normally, with the exception of a moderate elevation of the blood pressure.

How I Lost 36,000 Pounds

The patient was told that she was organically sound except for her obesity. The patient appeared to be a little cold, somewhat belligerent and suspicious. She had come for help because several of her friends had told her of the good results obtained in the treatment of obesity.

Mrs. E. consistently lost weight on the meat diet, combined with a weekly admonition that was almost a scolding from me. She continued to lose until I left for my vacation. During my absence she gained thirteen pounds. Her weight loss began again when we resumed regular conferences in which it was explained to her that the factors which made her gain weight in the first place were still operating and would cause further gain unless they were dealt with. These factors seemed to be a need for love and security which she had failed to find as a child and had sought but not found in her marriage.

Obviously, the role of the doctor is crucial in this weight loss, and it is doubtful if the patient can maintain her lower weight without the constant attention and reassurance of visits with her physician. It is apparent that in this case, the patient needs to understand or to eliminate the causes which contributed to her habitual overeating. This case further indicates the important truth that obesity is an unnatural state for man and has its roots in his emotional life. Some individuals, without digging out those roots, or even examining them, can reduce their weight and then maintain the loss, indicating a certain stability of personality which allows them to adopt a diet and then stick to it.

* * *

MRS. J. J. U., A THIRTY-YEAR-OLD HOUSEWIFE, MARRIED ten years with two living children, had been overweight for many years, saying that her usual weight was one hundred and eighty-five pounds. Mrs. U.'s case reveals the importance of motivation in the diet experience. She determined to reduce when she began to plan a trip, her first since her marriage, back to her parents' home in a distant State. She confided that she had always been made to feel inferior, and she was determined to show her family that in appearance, at least, she was superior.

Mrs. U. succeeded in transforming herself in a period of five months. Some individuals can be attractive in spite of obesity, but Mrs. U. was not one of these. When she began her diet, she was so discouraged about her weight that she was careless about her clothes, her hair, even about her fingernails. Five months later she had transformed herself into a truly beautiful woman with a weight of one hundred twenty-eight pounds. Her new

How I Lost 36,000 Pounds

appearance encouraged her to give more careful attention to other details of herself.

* * *

MRS. E., FIVE FEET SIX, A WOMAN OF RATHER SMALL bones, weighed 191 and one-half pounds; her husband weighed 196 pounds. Mr. E. was five feet eight inches tall and came in to reduce because of dizzy spells and a "nervous stomach." He was put on the meat diet and stayed on it without variation for four months. During this time he reduced to 156 pounds. His wife, Mrs. E., impressed by his success, then began a rigorous reducing schedule and during a period of eight months reduced to 127 pounds. Both Mr. and Mrs. E. have maintained their new weight.

* * *

MISS C. WEIGHED 196 AND ONE-HALF POUNDS AT SEVENteen years of age. She was a blond, attractive girl, valedictorian of her class in high school. Her father was also heavy, weighing about 275, although not obviously greatly overweight because he was very muscular. Miss C. was going with a boy whose mother was very fat and who constantly encouraged her to overeat.

Miss C. decided to reduce when she broke up with the boy she liked and wanted to get another date to attend

Cases

the senior prom. She picked out a small-sized frock in a dress shop as the dress she wanted to wear to the prom. Miss C.'s motives well illustrate the kind of thinking that often induces children and young people to begin a reducing diet.

Miss C. settled down, supposedly on the meat diet. She insisted that she was following this diet meticulously. Once when angry, however, she admitted that on some occasions she had substituted shrimp for the meat prescribed, although I had explained to her that no substitutions were to be used. Needless to say, until she made this admission, her weight loss was irregular. She did reduce to the size of the dress she had selected, and when she left for college she had reduced to 155 pounds.

* * *

MRS. D., 33, FIVE FEET NINE AND WITH THREE CHILDREN, weighed 235 and one-half pounds. She decided to reduce because of dizzy spells, stomach pains, and similar discomforts. Over a period of eight months she reduced to 156 and one-half pounds, a weight appropriate for her height and bone structure. About two years later she returned for a condition unrelated to diet and had gained almost up to her former weight. At that time she weighed 225 pounds. She dieted again until she weighed 207

How I Lost 36,000 Pounds

pounds and has since not appeared in the office. The lesson to be learned from this patient is that if the dieter regains his lost weight after his first heroic efforts to lose, it is twice as hard to lose a second time.

* * *

MR. B., A FORTY-YEAR-OLD MAN, WHO WAS SO HEAVY he could not be weighed on the scales, had been a heavyweight most of his life. He decided to reduce because of increasing poor health and feelings of weakness. His blood pressure was only a little above normal, and tests revealed that his feelings of ill health were not derived from any malfunctioning of glands or organs except for a mild heart strain and lungs that could hardly expand due to excess fat. In other words, his feelings of ill health were entirely due to his obesity. He was about six feet tall and weighed over 300 pounds.

From October of one year to July of the following year, this patient reduced to 177 pounds and has maintained this weight on the modified meat diet.